# Cure Herpes Naturally

## Natural Cures for a Herpes Free Life

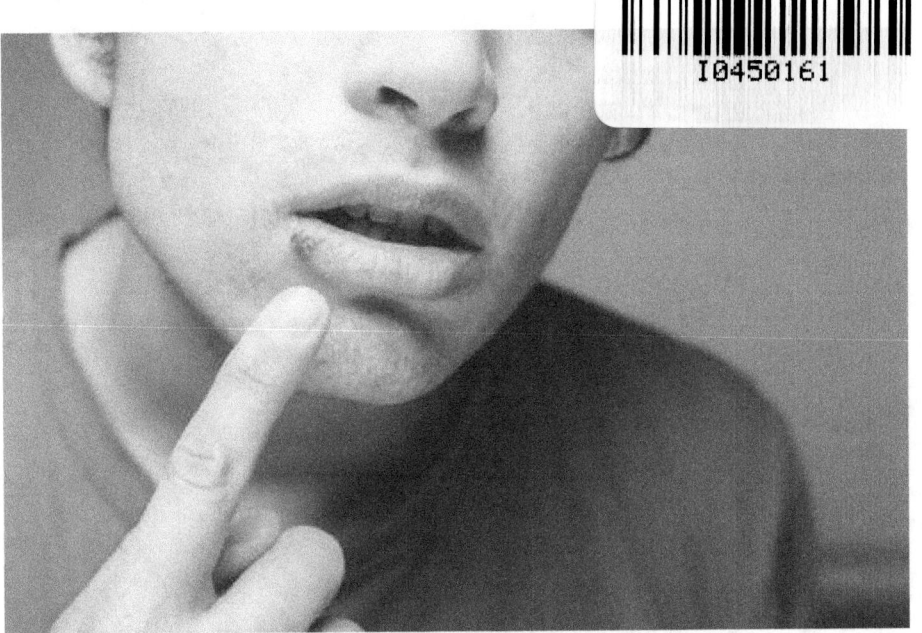

## Health Learning Series

M. Usman

Mendon Cottage Books

*JD-Biz Publishing*

**Disclaimer**

The information is this book is provided for informational purposes only. It is not intended to be used and medical advice or a substitute for proper medical treatment by a qualified health care provider. The information is believed to be accurate as presented based on research by the author.

The contents have not been evaluated by the U.S. Food and Drug Administration or any other Government or Health Organization and the contents in this book are not to be used to treat cure or prevent disease.

The author or publisher is not responsible for the use or safety of any diet, procedure or treatment mentioned in this book. The author or publisher is not responsible for errors or omissions that may exist.

**Warning**

The Book is for informational purposes only and before taking on any diet, treatment or medical procedure, it is recommended to consult with your primary health care provider.

Check out some of the other Healthy Gardening Series books at Amazon.com

Gardening Series on Amazon

Check out some of the other Health Learning Series books at Amazon.com

Health Learning Series on Amazon

# Table of Contents

# Introduction

A young man comes to his doctor and complains of painful sores around his genitals. During the inquiry the doctor finds out that he had unprotected sex with his partner while he was on vacation a month earlier. After a thorough examination the doctor concludes that he is suffering from a sexually transmitted disease (STD) called herpes.

Herpes is a sexually transmitted disease common in sexually active individuals. According to stats of the United States Center for Disease Control and Prevention (CDC), the reported cases of herpes are highest among any other sexually transmitted disease. According to the 2008 report of CDC, sexually transmitted diseases affect 19.7% of individuals in the United States per year. Herpes account for more than half of the reported cases of STDs. To be more precise, herpes affects more than 14 million individuals in the United States each year. Out of these cases most of the affected population (more than 49%) belongs to the age group of 15-24 years. The stats are truly alarming, right?

Whenever someone talks about sexually transmitted diseases, the first thing that comes to mind is AIDS. AIDS is a potentially lethal condition with no known cure. This leads to a misconception that whatever spreads through sex is supposed to be incurable and lethal. But this is not true. Although herpes can cause serious complications, it is not incurable. It can be diagnosed and treated with a 100% success rate.

What would you do if you get herpes? The first option that might come to mind, while suffering from a herpes infection, is going to a physician. But this is not a good choice because of two reasons. First, it's going to cost you A LOT. Second, you'll have to eat a handful of medicines each day and medicines have a lot of side effects ranging from minor to severe. "What other choice do I have then?" you might ask. Who needs to see a Doctor when all you need to do is search your kitchen or pantry or go to the super market for natural herpes cures? Confused? Read on to get your questions answered!

Here's some good news: You don't need to go to your Doctor and waste your time and money. There are natural methods that can do the trick for you. All these methods are cost effective, safe to use and guess what; you can try these methods all by yourself! Yes, home remedies, herbs, and natural cures have side effects too, but only if taken in high excess and if you don't follow the instructions or listen carefully or discuss these with your practitioner. This book will provide easy, achievable steps you can take, with none of the vague technical terms that won't help.

Read on to know everything you need to know about herpes, its origin, signs and symptoms and natural cures.

# Section 1: Getting Started

# Chapter 1: Herpes for dummies

Before we can jump to the natural cures for herpes, it would be better if you know some basics. Once you know what the problem is, solving it becomes much easier.

Herpes simplex or herpes is a viral disease. It is one of the most common sexually transmitted diseases (STDs). Although it most commonly spread through sex, it can also transfer from one person to another through direct contact (shedding of skin) and body fluids like blood, semen and vaginal fluid. Most commonly this disease affects genitals including the vagina, penis, anal area and buttocks, but it can include other parts of the body too like the mouth, eyes and even the brain.

Herpes, depending on its site of infection, can be divided into several sub types. How this infection presents is another topic and is discussed in the subsequent chapters. Depending on the site of infection, herpes can be divided into the following types:

| Site of infection. | Name of infection. |
|---|---|
| Tongue and gums | Herpetic gingivostomatitis |
| Lips | Herpes labialis |
| Genitals | Herpes genitalis |
| Fingers and thumbs | Herpetic whitlow. |
| Skin of face, ears and neck | Herpes gladiatorum. |
| Brain | Herpesviral encephalitis. |
| Food tube (esophagus) | Herpes esophagitis. |

This information might be a little too scientific for you but you need not worry. All you need to know at this point is what the different forms of herpes infection are. Herpes is not all about infection and cold sores on lips and genitals- as the misconceptions go. There are so many forms that herpes can take and treatment options vary with each form.

"I understand herpes and its types but what causes herpes in the first place?" this question might be popping into your mind at this point. Your question is excellent and here is the answer to your question. Herpes, as mentioned above, is a viral infection and is caused by the following viruses:

- Herpes simplex type 1 virus (HSV-1). This type of virus most commonly affects the face, eyes, throat, mouth and brain.
- Herpes simplex type 2 virus (HSV-2). This type of virus most commonly affects the anal region and genitals.

# Chapter 2: Who gets herpes infection?

Until now, you've read what herpes is and what causes herpes infection. But what makes you more prone to this infection? Is this infection age or gender related? All these questions will be answered in this chapter.

HSV-1 infection is most common among infants or children. Children mostly get this infection from infected adults that kiss or pinch their cheeks. The herpes virus travels from the skin of adults to the children (skin to skin transfer). To make it simple for you, children get herpes infection when they:

- Get a kiss.
- Are touched on the cheeks by an affected adult.
- Share kitchen utensils, like silverware, with the affected adults.
- Accidently cut themselves with sharp objects like razors contaminated with the virus.

Adults can also get HSV-1 infection and the reasons are the same as mentioned above.

HSV-2 infection, however, is very common among young adults that have unprotected sex. Age group of 15-24 years is most susceptible to get this infection because individuals belonging to this age group tend to have unprotected sex with multiple partners. The most important risk factors that make an individual at a higher risk to get HSV-2 infection include:

- Although this infection can target both males and females, the prevalence of HSV-2 infection is higher among females.
- Individuals having multiple sex partners are more likely to get this infection as compared to people that are tied to one partner.
- Unprotected sex is the most important cause of HSV-2 infection. Use of condoms significantly reduces the chances of spread of this infection.
- People that get sexually mature and active at a younger age are more likely to suffer from this infection.

- The chances of HSV-2 infection increase significantly if you've had some other sexually transmitted disease at some point during your life.
- Body has got an excellent immune system that stops foreign invaders like viruses from causing infection. Any reason that could weaken your immune system puts you more at risk to get this infection. Weakened immune system is most common among:
  - HIV sufferers.
  - Diabetics.
  - Patients suffering from cancers.
  - Individuals using immunosuppressant drugs.
  - Patients exposed to radiation therapy.

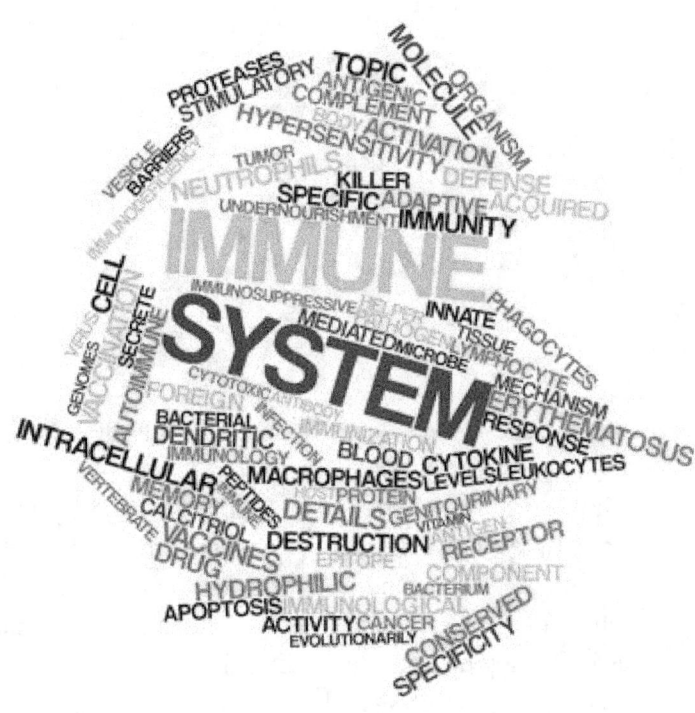

# Chapter 3: How to tell if you have herpes?

Most of the people who get herpes infection are asymptomatic i.e. they don't feel or experience anything at all. But, the other half of the people experience a number of symptoms including:

- **Sores.**

  The thing that people complain of the most when they get herpes is cold sores. These are one or more fluid filled blisters that might appear on different sites of the body depending on the type of herpes. These blisters burst, fluid oozes out of them and ultimately they turn into a thick crust before healing completely. These sores last for a time period of 7 to 10 days.

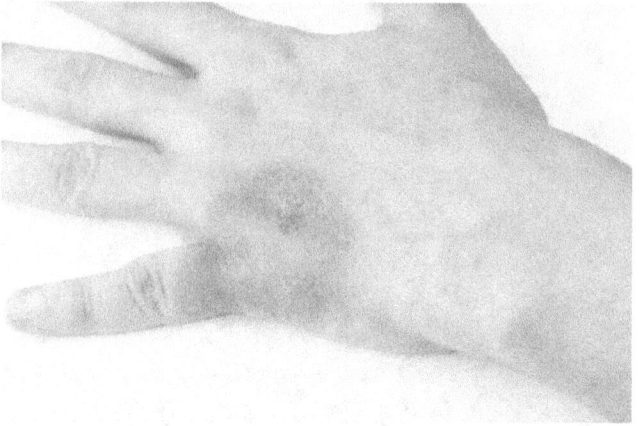

  The location of these sores depends on the variety of herpes:

  - Oral herpes (HSV-1):

    These sores usually develop on lips or around the mouth. Sometimes the affected areas also include inside of the mouth, gums and tongue. These are the most common areas where blisters are found in HSV-1 infection but blisters can also develop on any site on the skin.

  - Genital herpes (HSV-2):

    The sores in this case usually appear on or around the vagina, penis, buttocks and anal area. In some cases the affected women might develop sores inside the vagina. Although these are the most commonly affected areas in

HSV-2 infections, sores can also appear on multiple skin sites as in HSV-1 infection.

- **Itching, burning or tingling.**
Such sensations appear usually before the appearance of sores or blisters.

- **Flu like symptoms.**
These symptoms might appear with or without the appearance of sores. A generalized feeling of being ill (malaise), fever, cough, fatigue, muscle pain and enlarged lymph nodes (structures in the neck, groin) might also follow herpes infection.

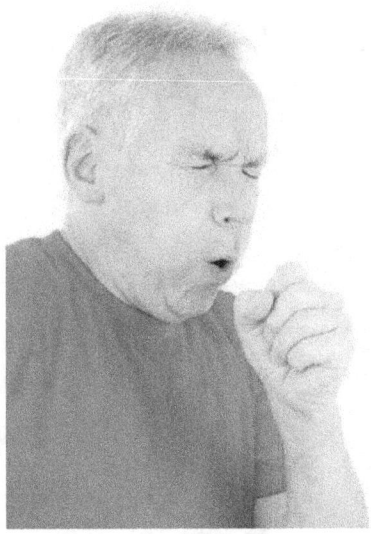

- **Burning during urinating.**
This problem is most common among the sufferers of genital herpes. The affected individual might find it difficult to pass urine or feel a painful, burning sensation while passing urine.

- **Eye infection**.
Eye infection is very common following oral and genital herpes. You might experience a gritty sensation in your eyes. You might

also experience sensitivity to light, discharge from your eye or generalized pain in your eyes.

# Section 2: How to cure herpes naturally?
# Chapter 4: Go Green, Go for herbs

Now that you know some basic information about herpes, its causes and most important, it's symptoms, we now move on to the basic topic of our book. Whenever anyone gets any disease or infection, the first choice is to go to a physician. But as discussed before, this method is costly and can have several side effects. The second choice that you have is to go for natural, herbal ways for treating herpes. These methods are extremely cost effective, have limited side effects, and you can readily try these methods at home, all by yourself. You don't need to be a healthcare professional to try these methods. Just follow the methods mentioned here and see the results for yourself.

Here is a compilation of several herbal ways that have helped so many people in getting rid of herpes infection. Here is your complete guide to the herbal ways to cure herpes, how these ways work and some precautions that you must observe to avoid any unnecessary side effects.

### *How to cure herpes sores?*

## Lemon balm (*Melissa officinalis*)

**What?** Lemon balm, also known as *Melissa officinalis,* is a plant belonging to the family of mint. This herb has been used since prehistoric times and is considered to produce a calming effect on the body. This herb can also be used for the treatment of insomnia, anxiety, bee stings and also has antimicrobial activity.

One of the biggest problems that people want to get rid of, when they get herpes infection, is herpes sores. These sores pose a cosmetic problem and seriously shiver the confidence of an individual. Lemon balm has been found extremely effective in curing the cold sores associated with herpes infection. In one study, 116 people with herpes infection were asked to apply lemon balm on the sores on their skin. Most of the people reported significant reduction in the redness and swelling associated with herpes sores even within 2 days after they started using lemon balm. [1][2]

**How?** Topical application forms of lemon balm are easily available. Apply this balm on the affected sites 2-3 times a day or as per recommended.

**Caution** Topical forms of lemon balm are very safe to use with limited side effects. If you have some pre-existing skin allergies then consult your health care provider before using lemon balm as it might cause exacerbation of a skin allergy.

## Aloe (*Aloe Vera*)

**What?** Aloe Vera is a plant growing in tropical regions of Latin America, Africa, and the Caribbean. This herb has been used since prehistoric times for the treatment of wounds, burns, irritation and constipation.

As far as the treatment of herpes sores is concerned, Aloe Vera is scientifically proven to decrease them. Aloe Vera gel can significantly reduce the symptoms of genital herpes. In one study it was found that application of Aloe Vera gel can significantly reduce the swelling associated with herpes sore and can also speed up the process of healing. [1][3]

**How?** One way to obtain Aloe Vera gel is to slit the leaf of Aloe Vera length wise and collect the gel from inside of the plant. If this method is too cumbersome for you then you can use the commercial preparations of this gel. Apply this gel generously on the affected areas 1-2 times each day. Make sure not to apply this gel on the open wounds.

**Caution** Aloe Vera gel is very safe to use. However, it shouldn't be applied on open or deep wounds as it can trigger an allergy.

## Rhubarb cream (*Rheum palmatum*)

**What?** This plant is found in several parts of the world including China, India, Turkey and Russia. The underground part of this herb is used for making medicines. This herb is used for the treatment of a number of gastrointestinal complications including diarrhea, constipation, hemorrhoids and stomach pain.

A Swiss study was conducted to see the efficiency of Rhubarb cream for the treatment of cold sores associated with herpes. Results showed that topical application of a mixture of this cream and sage extract is as effective as any other medicine used for the similar purpose. [1]

**How?** For the treatment of cold sores, use a cream containing 23 gm extract of Rhubarb and Sage extract. Apply this cream on the affected areas every 3-4 hours while awake. Continue with this treatment for one week or more until the symptoms abate.

**Caution** This cream is not safe for children as they might ingest it. The only side effect seen with the topical application of this cream is skin irritation.

## Melaleuca alternifolia (Tea Tree) Oil

**What?** Tea tree oil is derived from the leaves of *Melaleuca alternifolia*. Don't confuse tree tea with the tea plants used for making black or green herbal teas. This essential oil is used for treating a wide variety of fungal, bacterial and viral infections.

Some studies have shown that application of tea tree oil on the affected areas of the skin can help in the cure and management of herpes cold sores. The oral preparations of this oil are also helpful in the eradication of herpes virus from the body. [4]

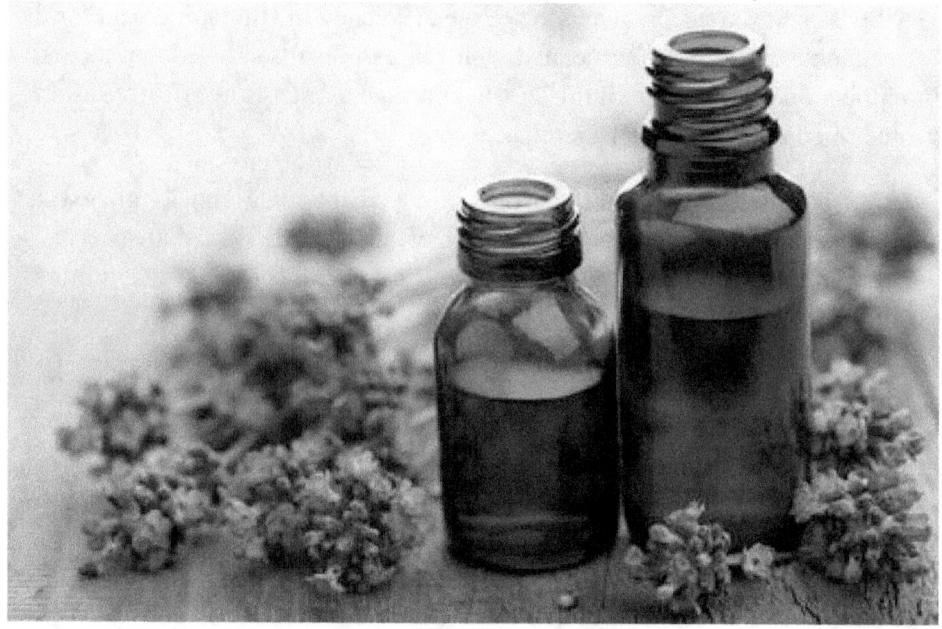

**How?** Use 6% tea tree oil for application on the cold sores. For 2-3 grams of tea tree dilute it in 150-200 ml of water. Apply this oil gently on the affected areas twice daily until the issue is resolved.

**Caution** Use of tea tree oil is not recommended for young boys that have not yet reached puberty, as it can cause hormonal imbalance is boys that might trigger the development of gynecomastia (male breasts). Moreover, people having some kind of skin irritation or skin allergy should only use tea tree oil after the recommendation of their health care provider.

## Eucalyptus Oil

**What?** Eucalyptus is a tree native to Asian countries like Pakistan and India. Eucalyptus oil is derived from the leaves of this tree. This amazing tree is used in the treatment of hundreds of ailments including gastrointestinal disorders, tuberculosis, mononucleosis, cancer, acne, asthma, ring worm infections, skin infections and so on.

Eucalyptus oil is available in the form of both oral and topical preparations. Oral preparations of eucalyptus oil are used for the treatment of herpes infection as a whole. The topical application of eucalyptus oil is a proven remedy for herpes cold sores. [4]

**How?** Take some leaves of eucalyptus and rub them with your palms. You'll see a fluid oozing out of the leaves. You can apply this gently on your sores. But, this method is cumbersome and you might not get it right, so the better way is to use the preparations of Eucalyptus oil that are easily available in the market. The concentration of Eucalyptus oil used depends on age, sex and general health. For an average adult 5-20% concentration can be used for topical application. 0.2-0.3 gm of eucalyptus oil when applied on the skin can do the trick. If your skin is sensitive, you can dilute it in a few teaspoons of water. Apply this solution on the affected area 2-3 times a day for a week.

**Caution** You have to be very careful about the concentration and amount of eucalyptus oil used. Concentrated forms of eucalyptus oil, even when applied on the skin in a very small amount, can cause severe skin reactions, pain, redness, and itching. Also, you need to be very careful about the amount of this oil used. Small amounts of oil might not do any harm, but large amounts of oil, even when diluted, can trigger skin allergies.

## Peppermint oil

**What?** This essential oil is derived from the peppermint plant. This plant is most commonly found in North America and Europe. Peppermint oil is used in the treatment of a number of ailments including irritable bowel syndrome, heartburn, indigestion, nausea, vomiting, common cold, menstrual abnormalities and headache. A research was conducted in the University of Heidelberg, Germany where researchers evaluated the efficacy of the peppermint oil when used for the treatment of herpes infection. Results were very promising and it was found that peppermint oil can treat both infection of herpes and herpes sores. [5]

**How?** Apply 1 drop of 10% peppermint oil on the site of sore and rub gently with the help of a cotton swab. Repeat this process 1-2 times a day for 1 week. Individuals with sensitive skin can dilute this oil before use.

**Caution** Usually this oil is very safe to use but some individuals might develop skin flushes and allergic reactions when the oil is applied directly to the skin without dilution. Make sure to use appropriate dilution of peppermint oil.

### *How to eradicate herpes from within?*

Until now we've discussed the treatment options for herpes cold sores. Although cold sores are only a minor problem associated with herpes, for most of the people, treating cold sores gains more importance since it poses a major cosmetic threat- this is understandable as well. So, now that you know how to treat the sores of herpes, we now move on to discuss several ways through which herpes virus can be eradicated from within.

Here is a list of herbs that are scientifically proven to possess an anti-viral activity and can be used to treat herpes virus from within.

## Siberian ginseng

**What?** Serbian ginseng is a plant that the root is used for making several medicines. This magical herbal plant is used for the treatment of hundreds of ailments including high blood pressure, arthritis, diabetes and respiratory diseases.

A research was conducted on 93 sufferers of herpes infection over a period of 6 months where they ingested this herb. Results were promising and showed that the use of this herb significantly reduces the duration, intensity and frequency of herpes infection. [1] Ginseng is particularly very effective for the treatment of type 2 herpes infection.

**How?** For the treatment of HSV-2 infection, ginseng preparations are taken by mouth. For the treatment of genital herpes ginseng extract is mixed with eleutheroside E 0.3% to make 400mg daily dosage.

**Caution** Make sure to take ginseng according to the recommended dosage. Consuming too much ginseng can trigger a number of side effects including drowsiness, abnormal heart rhythm, anxiety and high blood pressure. Use of this herb is particularly contraindicated in pregnant and breast feeding females, people with heart diseases, and people with breast cancer.

# Cinnamon

**What?** It is a plant that the bark and flowers are used for making medicines. It is used for the treatment of a variety of ailments including high blood pressure, gastrointestinal disturbance, and diabetes.

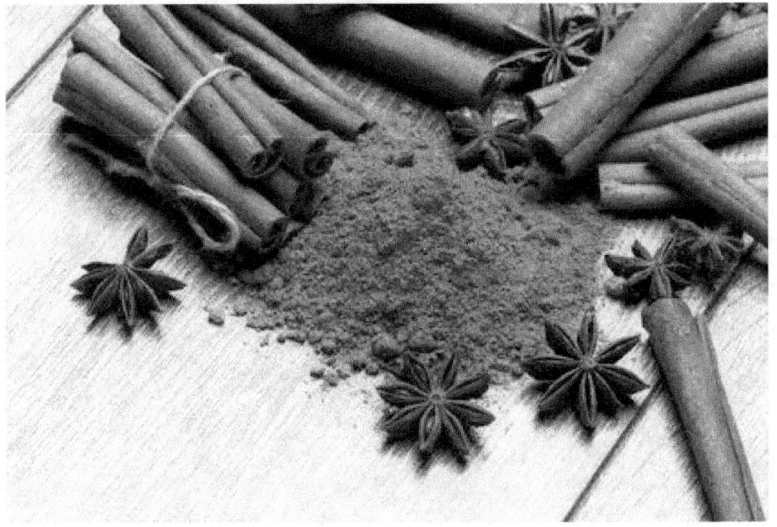

A research was conducted in The University of Tokyo where researchers found that certain chemicals present in the bark of cinnamon have strong anti-viral activity. Those chemicals were collected, purified and were tested against type 1 herpes virus. Results showed that cinnamon extract has strong anti-herpes properties. [6]

**How?** Cinnamon supplements are available but the exact dosage depends on age, sex and health status. One very safe way to consume cinnamon for the cure of herpes infection is by making cinnamon tea. For this purpose heat 1 cup of water until it boils. Add 1-2 teaspoons of cinnamon powder in this water and heat for a few more minutes. Strain the liquid and add 1 teaspoon of honey in this liquid to make it taste good. Drink this healthful tea 1-2 times a day.

**Caution** Pregnant and breast feeding females should avoid the use of cinnamon. Moreover people with diabetes, liver disease or people that have to undergo some surgery should be careful while using cinnamon. Otherwise cinnamon, in the form of tea, is very safe to use.

## Allium sativum (garlic)

**What?** Garlic is a plant that is best known for flavoring food. This kitchen ingredient has long been used for the treatment of hundreds of ailments. Garlic is particularly effective for the treatment of blood pressure, high cholesterol, heart diseases, acne and several forms of cancer.

A research conducted in the Brigham Young University, USA proved that garlic extracts are extremely effective in the treatment of a number of viral infections including both type 1 and type 2 herpes infections. [7]

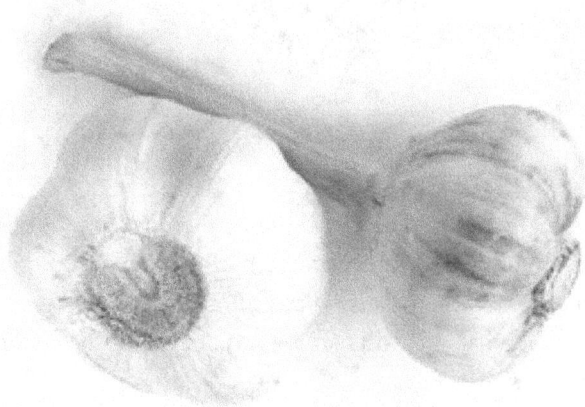

**How?** 2.91mg/ml and 3.05mg/ml (2.91mg in 1ml water and 3.05 in 1ml water) is the proven concentration for the cure of herpes infection.

**Caution** Overuse of garlic extracts can trigger allergic reactions, bleeding disorders and gastrointestinal upset. Moreover, use of this extract is contraindicated in pregnant and breastfeeding females and patients with bleeding disorders and stomach ulcers.

# Ginger (Zingiber officinale)

**What?** Some say ginger is an herb; others say it's a spice. Whatever it is, it is extremely beneficial for the treatment of a variety of ailments. It can be used fresh, in the form of oil, or in dried form. It is commonly used for the treatment of gastrointestinal distress, high blood pressure, diabetes, aches and pains, and airway problems. A research was conducted in which some herbs were tested for their activity against type 1 herpes infection. Researchers concluded that extracts of ginger are extremely effective in killing type 1 herpes virus. [8] Some studies also support the efficacy of the use of ginger for the treatment of type 2 herpes. [9]

**How?** The daily consumption of ginger, in any form, should not exceed 4gm. 500mg capsules of ginger extracts are available that can be eaten twice a day. Another way to use ginger is by making a tea. For this purpose take a few inches piece of ginger and peel off its skin. Chop this ginger into fine pieces. Take 1-2 cups of water and add these chopped pieces into the water. Heat water until it boils. Strain the liquid and let it cool down a bit. Add honey to improve the taste of this liquid. Consume this liquid 2-3 times a day.

**Caution** Overuse of ginger tincture, capsules or tea can trigger severe stomach upset, nausea, vomiting and diarrhea. It might also increase the susceptibility of bleeding in some individuals. The use of ginger is contraindicated in pregnant, breast feeding females and individuals with heart disease and bleeding disorders.

# Echinacea pallida

<u>What?</u> This is an herb that the leaves, roots and flowers are used for the preparation of medicines. This herb is used for the treatment of cold, urinary tract infection and variety of bacterial and viral infections.

There is a mixed view regarding if this herb really works in curing herpes infection. But, most of the studies do suggest that the extract of this herb can cure herpes infection. One such research was conducted at the University of Heidelberg, Germany, which showed that extracts derived from Echinacea pallida have significant anti-HSV-1 and HSV-2 activity. [10]

**How?** Specific capsule preparations of this herb are available and taking 800 mg capsules twice a day might help eradicate herpes infection.

**Caution** Overuse of this herb can trigger gastrointestinal upset, dizziness, muscle and joint pains. This herb should particularly be avoided in children as it can trigger allergic reactions in them. Moreover, the use of this herb is contraindicated in pregnant and breast feeding females. Also, the use of this herb requires caution in those individuals that suffer some sort of autoimmune disorder like rheumatoid arthritis and systemic lupus erythematosus.

## St. John's Wort (Hypericum perforatum)

**What?** St. John's Wort is an herb that the flowers and leaves are used for making a number of medicines. This herb is used for the treatment of a number of disorders including anxiety, depression, joint pains, abnormal menstruation and fibromyalgia.

A number of biologically active ingredients are found in this herb, the most important of which is hypericin. Research has shown that hypericin has significant anti-viral activity against herpes virus. [11]

**How?** Never start or give up this herb without consulting your healthcare provider as it might trigger some serious side effects. The exact dose depends on age, sex and health condition. Generally 300-500 mg of the dose taken 3 times a day for 4-6 months is recommended for the treatment of a variety of ailments.

**<u>Caution</u>** St. John's Wort is a very tricky herb. When used according to the prescription and within given limits, it can do wonders for your health. But, if you don't follow instructions and use it excessively, you might end up facing some serious side effects. Side effects range from minor stomach upset to severe mental impairments. The use of this herb is contraindicated in pregnant, breast feeding, and patients with bipolar disorder, infertility issues, ADHD, Alzheimer's disease and schizophrenia.

# Chapter 5: Look before you eat!

The food we eat has a great impact on our overall health. Diseases are more prevalent now than they were ever before, because of the food we eat. If you ask someone what they like to eat the answer would surely be hamburgers, sausages, fried chips, pizzas and colas. These foods are nothing but bouts of bad sugar, cholesterol and fat. All these ingredients are harbingers of several health complications and weakened immune system. And people with weak immune systems, as mentioned before, are more likely to suffer from herpes infections. So look before you eat!

## Don't eat/Drink it!

Whatever you do, don't eat the below mentioned food before, during or after herpes infection. The basic idea here is to skip these foods because these foods weaken the immune system.

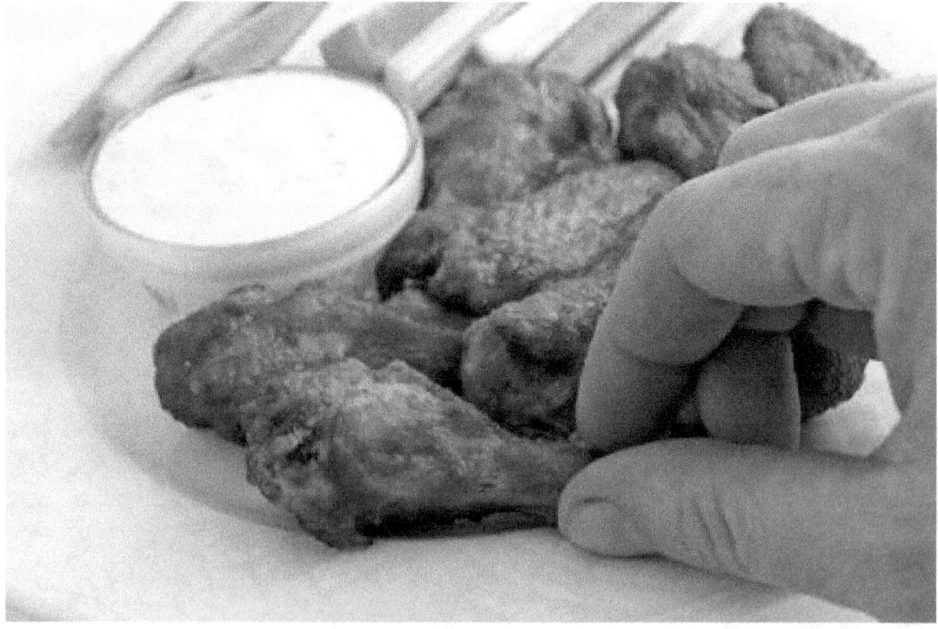

The foods that you should avoid include:

- All sorts of fried food should be avoided. Restrict the intake of animal fats.
- Avoid the consumption of all sorts of junk food including burgers, fries and sausages.
- Limit the intake of carbonated beverages.
- Put a stop to alcohol consumption.
- Don't smoke cigarettes.
- Don't eat processed or ready to eat foods.

## Eat/Drink it!

Increase the intake of following food items:

- Yogurt as it is rich in probiotics.
- Carrots.
- Nuts and seeds.
- Salmon and other seafood.
- Berries and plums.
- Sweet potatoes.

Following food supplements are also proven to cure herpes infections:

- **Lysine:** Lysine is an amino acid. Eating as much as 1-3 g of lysine each day can help during herpes infection. Research has shown the lysine can help in the healing of cold sores. Moreover, it can also reduce the intensity and frequency of herpes infection. [1] The best way to get lysine is from natural sources including fish, chicken, eggs and potatoes. However, you can add more lysine by eating lysine supplements.
- **Zinc:** Zinc is a mineral normally present in the body and is meant for regulating a number of chemical reactions in the body. Zinc is useful in treating both the sores and infection from within. In a research, scientists found that the application of zinc oxide cream on cold sores can speed up the recovery and healing. Moreover, other studies have shown that eating supplements having lysine and zinc can help manage symptoms of herpes. [1]

- **Propolis**: Propolis can be taken as a dietary supplement. It is a resin made by honey bees and is loaded with flavonoids (substances with anti-oxidant properties). It also helps in curing cold sores of herpes. Application of 3% ointment on the affected areas can help cure herpes sores. [1]

# Conclusion

Herpes is an infection that most commonly spreads through sexual contact with the affected person. Prevention is better than cure, they say and it holds true in the case of herpes as well. If you're vigilant enough to follow the guidelines of protected sex, you'll never catch this infection.

Things don't always go according to the plan, so it is better to know how to cure herpes infection. One choice that you have is to go to your doctor and spend a lot of your time and money for curing this ailment. Second option is to go for natural ways. We don't claim that herbal ways are without side effects. Yes, herbs have side effects too but only when they're misused. Herbs, however, are extremely cost effective and are easy to use. The side effects are limited and all the side effects and contra-individuations have been discussed in detail.

Here we're, towards the end of the book. What are you waiting for? If you have herpes and you're too ashamed to go to your doctor or tell your family or friend about this sexually transmitted disease, then you better start using the herbal ways mentioned in this book.

Hope the methods mentioned in this book help!

# References:

1.  http://umm.edu/health/medical/altmed/condition/herpes-simplex-virus
2.  http://umm.edu/health/medical/altmed/herb/lemon-balm
3.  http://umm.edu/health/medical/altmed/herb/aloe
4.  http://www.ncbi.nlm.nih.gov/pmc/articles/PMC1360273/
5.  http://www.ncbi.nlm.nih.gov/pubmed/13678235
6.  http://www.ncbi.nlm.nih.gov/pubmed/18089742
7.  http://www.ncbi.nlm.nih.gov/pubmed/1470664
8.  http://www.ncbi.nlm.nih.gov/pmc/articles/PMC1855548/
9.  http://www.ncbi.nlm.nih.gov/pubmed/17976968
10. http://www.ncbi.nlm.nih.gov/pubmed/19790030
11. http://www.ncbi.nlm.nih.gov/books/NBK92750/

# Author Bio

Muhammad Usman is a distinguished medical graduate of Allama iqbal medical college (AIMC). He is a professional writer who has been in the field for more than 4 years. During this time he has produced 10,000+ articles, blogs and eBooks on various niches related to diseases, health, fitness, nutrition and well-being. He is a regular contributor to several journals related to medicine and surgery. He is the editor of several journals and newspapers.

# Check out some of the other JD-Biz Publishing books

## Gardening Series on Amazon

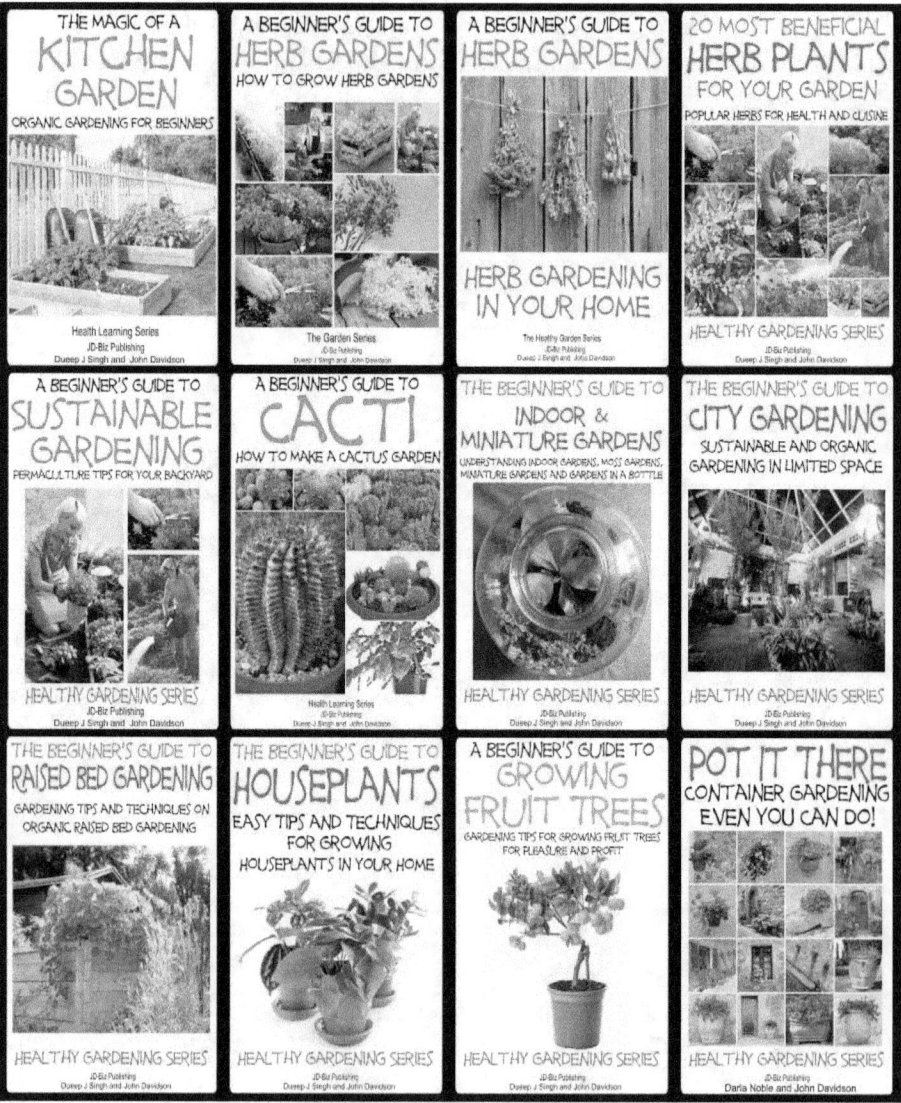

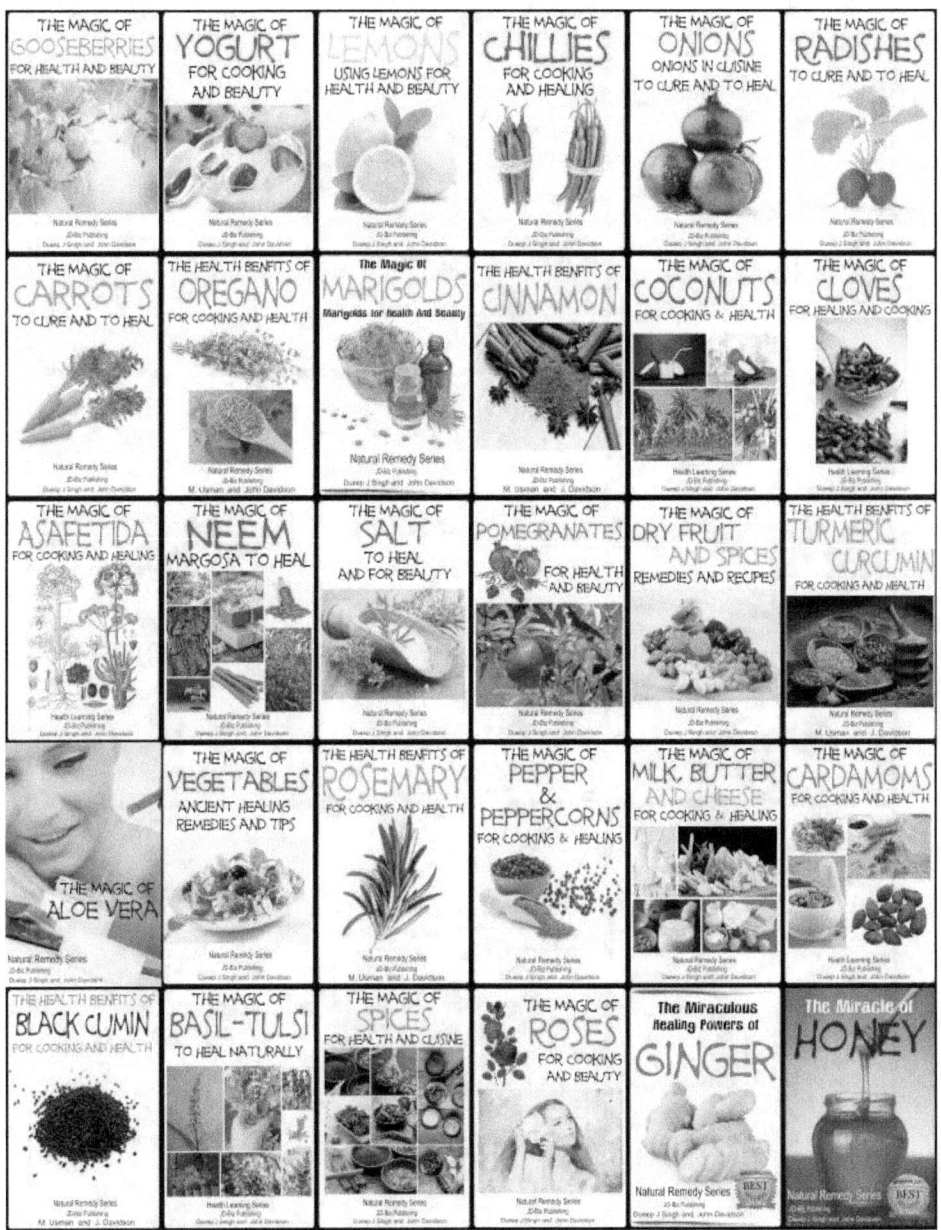

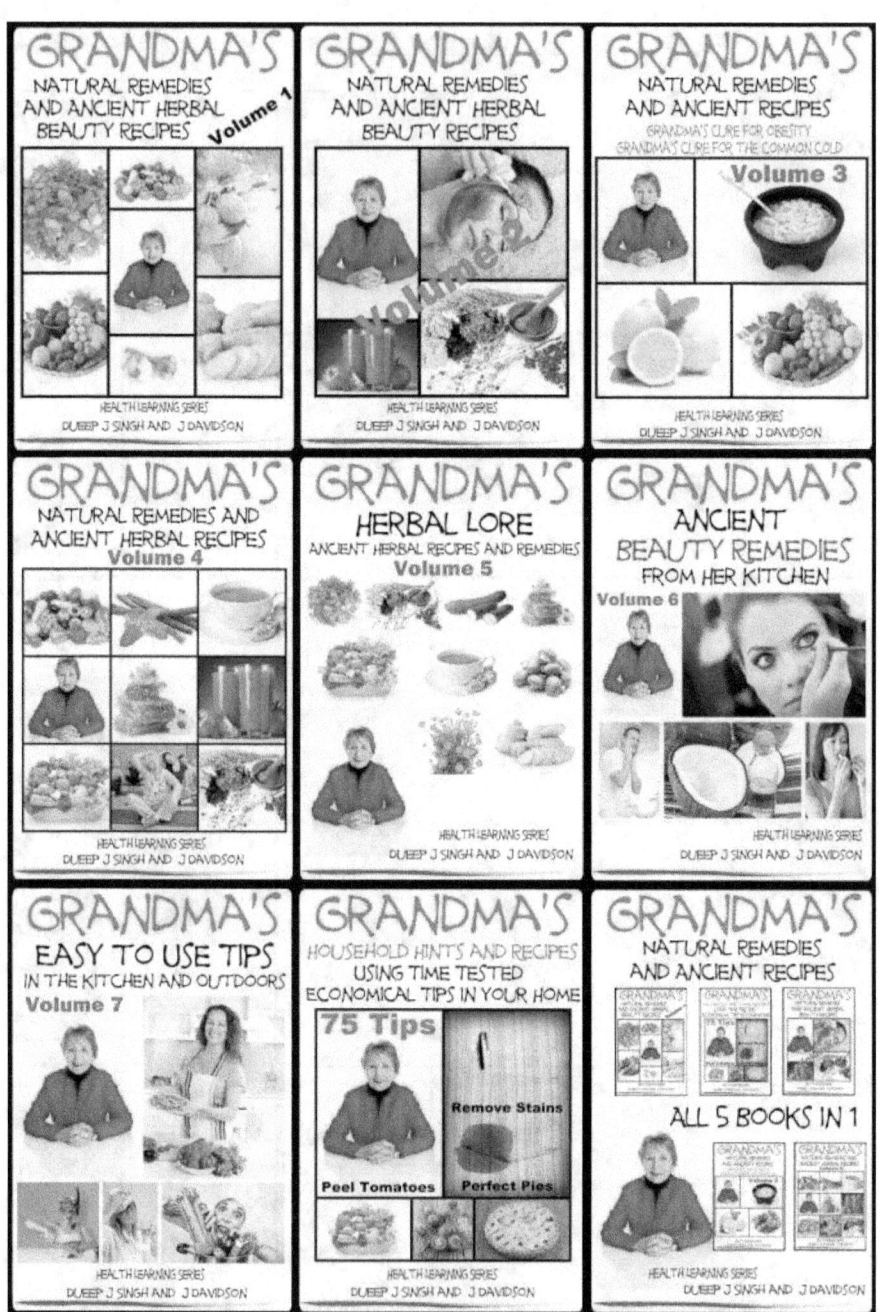

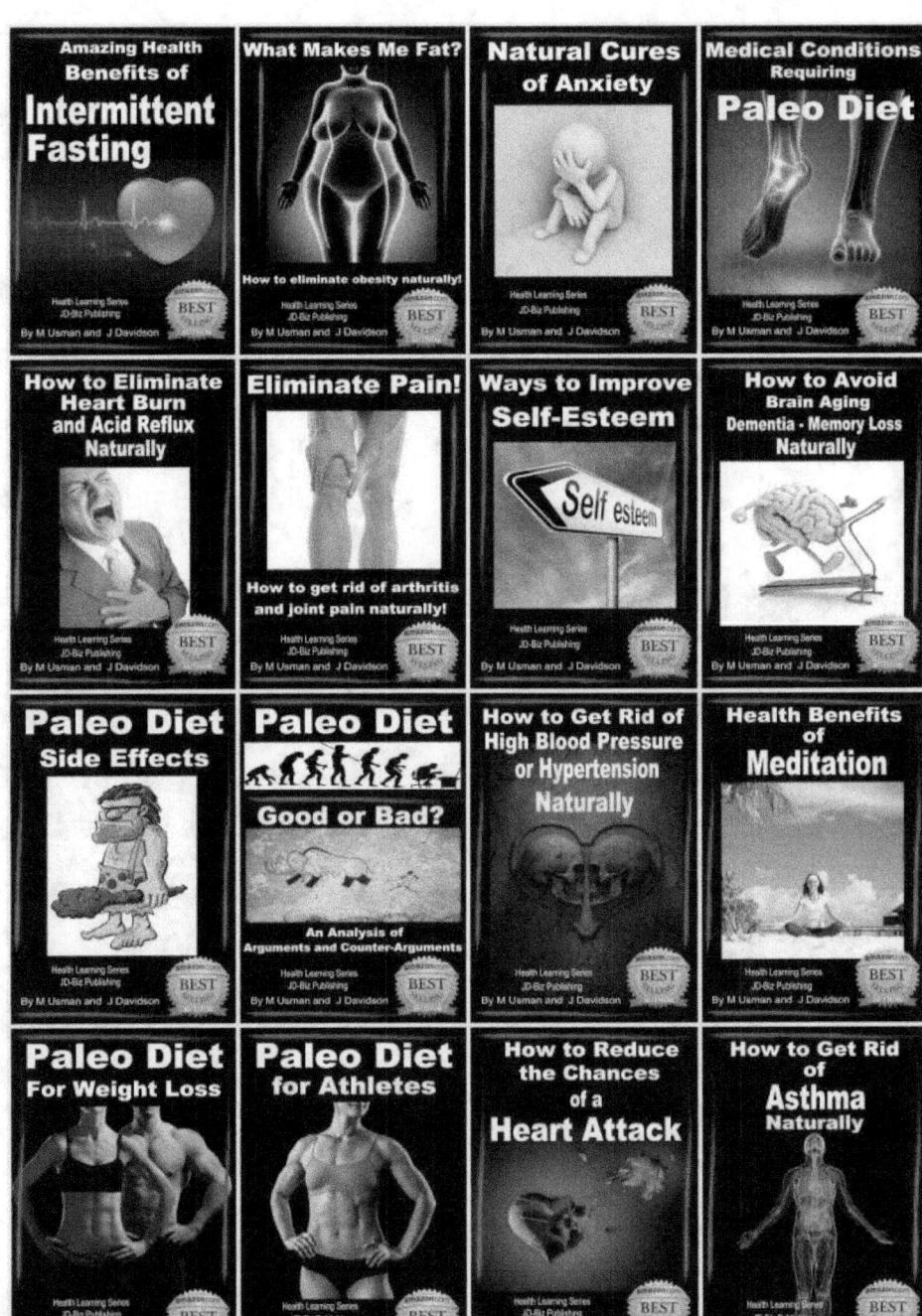

# Amazing Animal Book Series

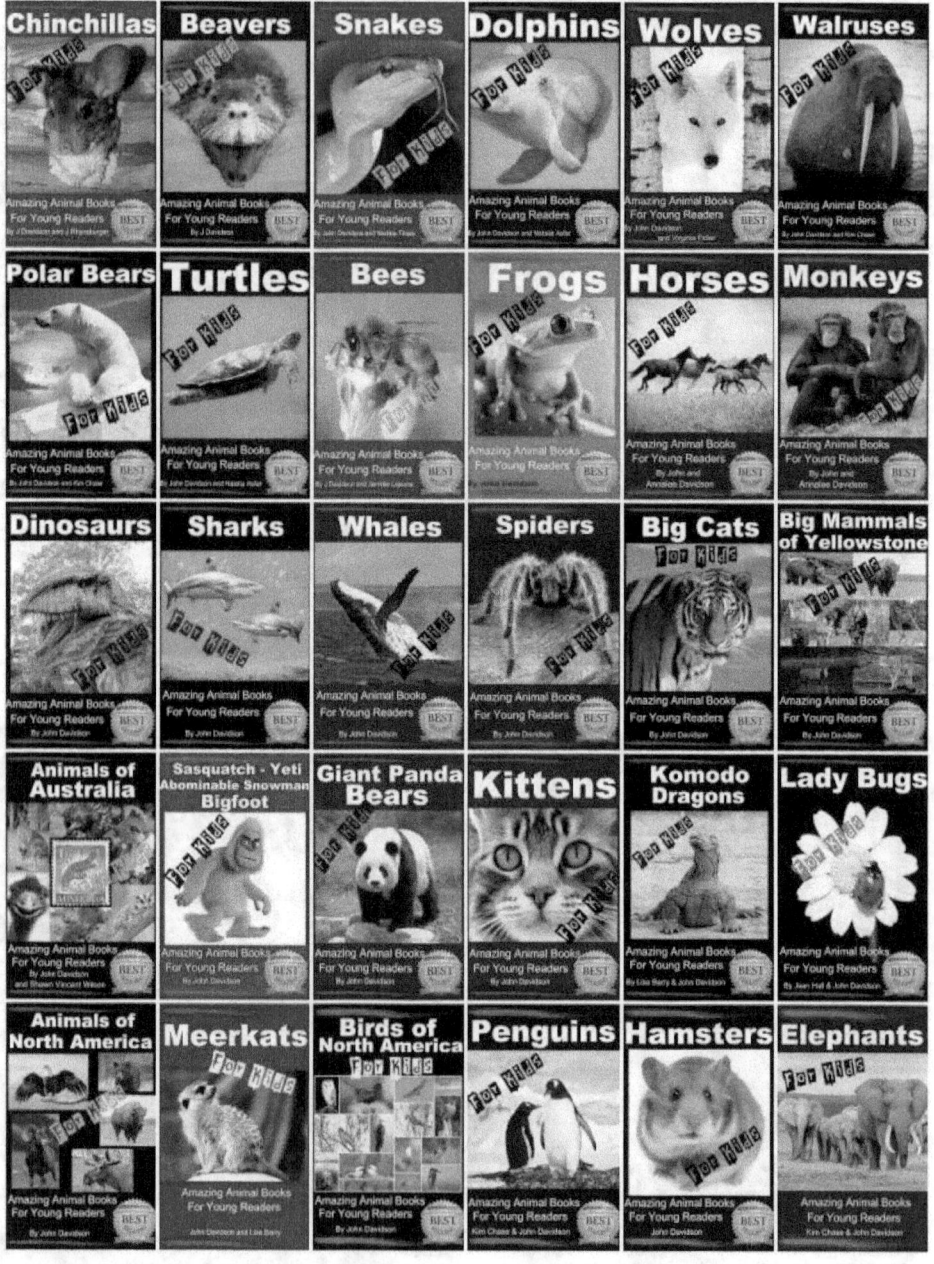

# Learn To Draw Series

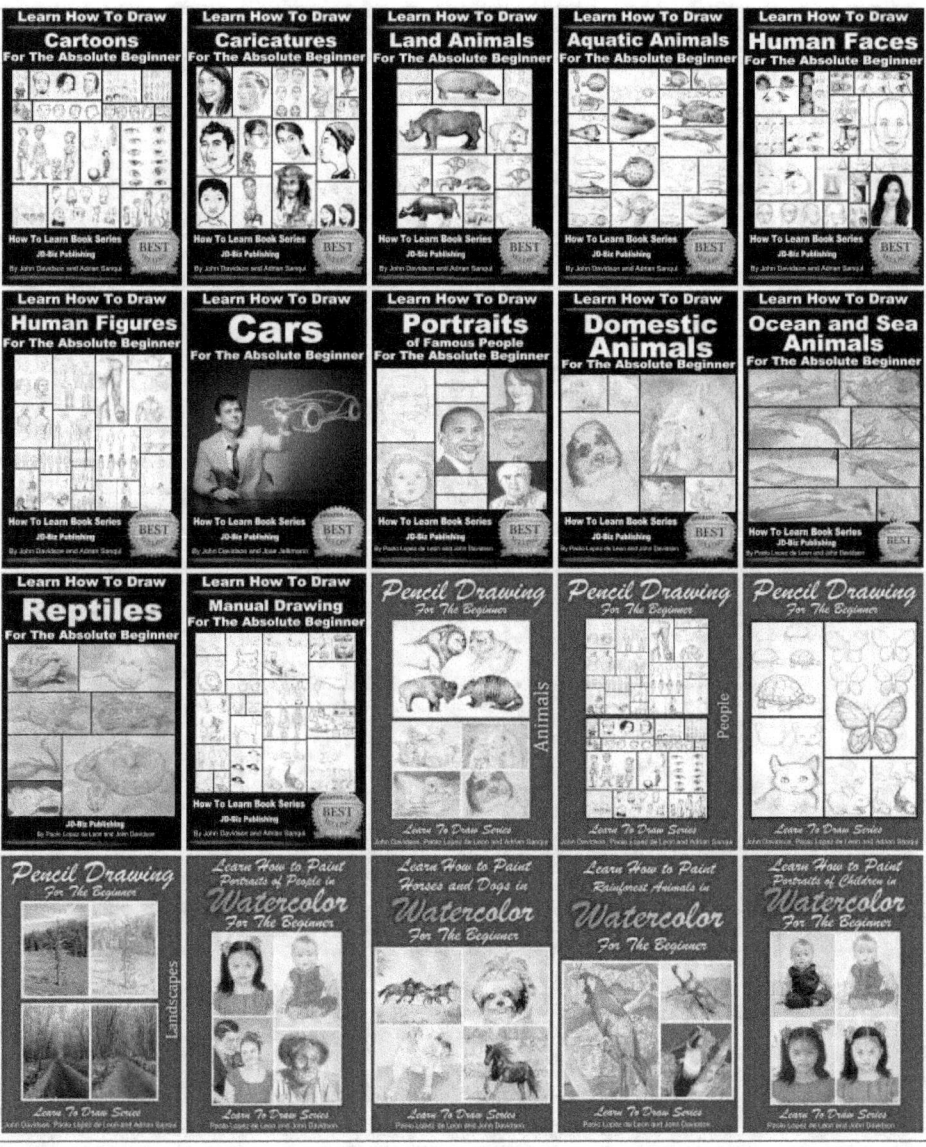

# How to Build and Plan Books

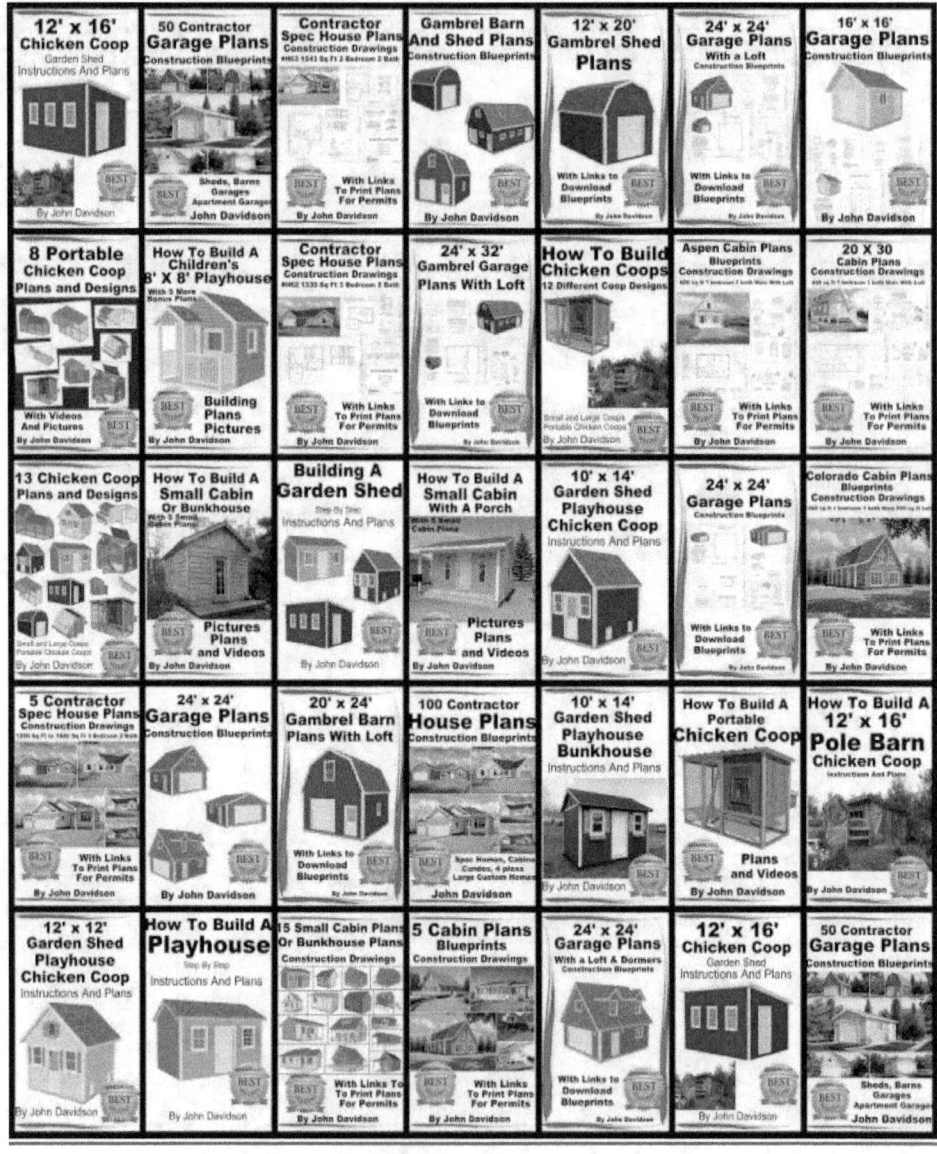

# Entrepreneur Book Series

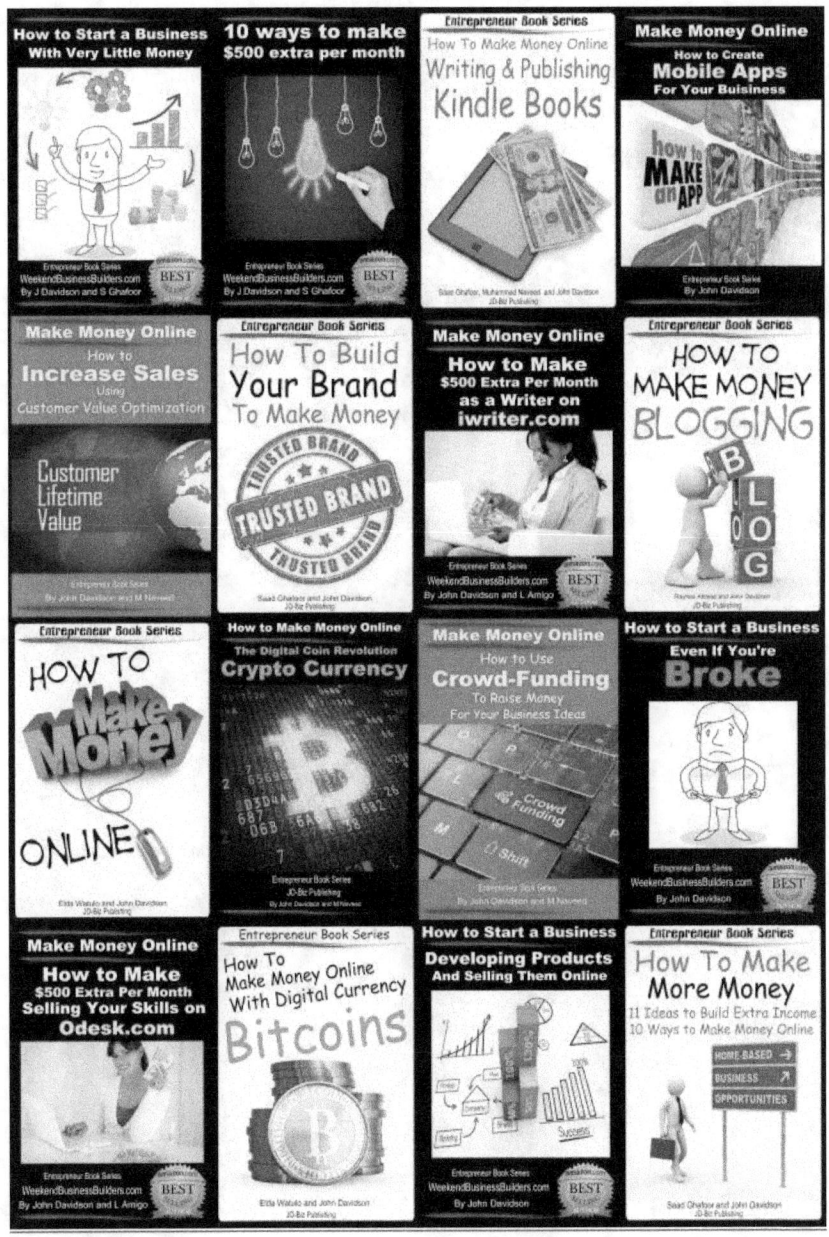

Our books are available at

1. Amazon.com

2. Barnes and Noble

3. Itunes

4. Kobo

5. Smashwords

6. Google Play Books

This book is published by

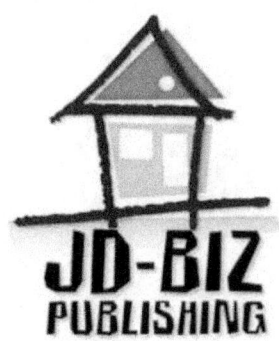

JD-Biz Corp

P O Box 374

Mendon, Utah 84325

http://www.jd-biz.com/

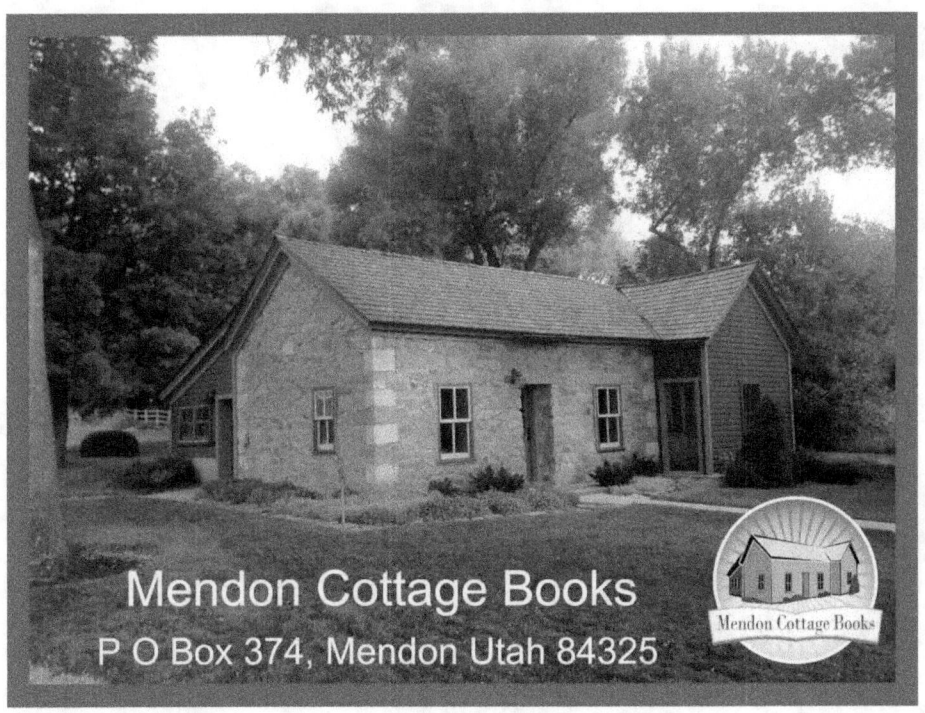

www.ingramcontent.com/pod-product-compliance
Lightning Source LLC
Chambersburg PA
CBHW061930280526
45787CB00004B/1551